How to Increase Your Energy Naturally

Linda Tremer

ISBN-10: 1508500231
ISBN-13: 978-1508500230

CONTENTS

CHAPTER 1- LIFE STYLE CHANGES

Introduction

Fatigue is one of the most common medical complaints.

"There are over 10 million visits per year to the primary care provider for problems relating to fatigue, with approximately 50% of the U.S. population reporting being fatigued for at least part of the day." (1)

It has been reported that over 20% of adults have severe fatigue. If you have fatigue and a lack of energy get a complete physical exam from your physician to rule out any illnesses.

Fatigue can come from many different causes. Everything from immune disorders, food allergies, environmental allergies, diabetes, blood sugar problems, metabolic disorder, obesity, infection, heart disease, cancer, fibromyalgia and menopause can cause fatigue and a lack of energy.

To combat fatigue, exhaustion, low energy and even brain fog there are many natural non toxic remedies. Some of these work for some people and others work for other people. Sometimes it's trial and error to find the right combination for you.

Once you have had a check up by your physician and ruled out any illness, you can try one of these natural solutions to increase your energy.

We will start our journey to eliminate fatigue with lifestyle changes. We will then discuss the vitamins and minerals that are vital in fighting fatigue. This is followed by herbal remedies that relieve fatigue. The section on nutraceuticals includes some cutting edge supplements that are being studied.

The next chapter details the importance of detoxifying your body. Miscellaneous supplements and other natural therapies are included. And finally there is a five step program to show you exactly what you need to do to eliminate your fatigue and increase your energy.

Many of you will be tempted to skip chapter one lifestyle changes and go right to chapters 4 and 7. I urge you to read and pay attention to chapter one because without life style changes fatigue will always be a part of your life.

Make Lifestyle Changes

The first step in combating fatigue is to make lifestyle

changes.

Lifestyle changes are the most important way to increase your energy. Simple changes in your life can really help you fight fatigue and feel more energized throughout the day.

So, what are these lifestyle changes that you can do in order to treat fatigue?

Change Your Diet

You can boost your physical and mental energy by eating a well-balanced diet. Nutritious foods are needed to create energy. Focus on eating organic fruits and vegetables, low fat dairy products, lean organic grass fed meats, and whole grain foods.

You have to reduce the amount of fat, sugar, and salt in your diet as well as your alcohol and caffeine intake. Empty foods like simple sugars, white flour and processed foods will sap your energy.

Stay away from sugary cereals, juices and caffeinated drinks. They can make you feel sluggish later in the day. Don't skip meals. Try to eat every 3 hours to keep your blood sugar levels up.

Let me briefly explain the role of insulin and fat. Insulin is a hormone produced by the pancreas. Insulin's role in the body is to regulate blood sugar (glucose levels). Insulin helps the glucose molecules enter the cells to provide energy. If your cells are sensitive to insulin the glucose is sent into your cells without any trouble and all is well.

Now here's where the trouble begins. The more carbohydrates you eat, the more glucose you will produce. Blood sugar levels rise rapidly when you eat refined carbohydrates. The body produces large amounts of insulin to deal with the excess glucose.

That increase in insulin in the blood stream causes the cells to lose their ability to respond to insulin. This is called insulin resistance.

Insulin resistance comes from eating refined carbohydrates, processed foods or too many calories.

Let me simplify it a bit more. When you eat a lot of processed foods you get a lot of glucose in your blood stream.

Your body keeps producing insulin because there is so much glucose in the blood stream but the glucose can't get into your cells since they have become resistant to all that insulin.

Without glucose your cells can't produce the energy you need.

Fatigue is one of the most common characteristics of insulin resistance. The condition can deplete your energy, leaving you exhausted. Other symptoms include fatigue, mental fatigue, and drowsiness after eating.

Excess insulin also keeps the fat that is already in the cells from being released for use as energy.

The standard American diet is low in fiber, and high in processed foods such as cookies, carbs, pasta, cake, soda, cereals, fried foods, high fructose corn syrup and simple sugars. These will cause your insulin levels to spike.

Eat good fats and high protein foods to keep your blood sugar from spiking.

Start eating more fresh fruits and vegetables. Make them the focus of your meals. Eat whole grains. Consume baked not fried foods. Eat more raw foods. Eat lean protein instead of fatty foods. Choose organic whenever possible. Do not consume genetically modified foods.

Artificial chemicals and sweeteners can also cause fatigue.

Gluten

More and more professional athletes are giving up gluten. Some have celiac disease but others have found that a gluten free diet helps their performance, stamina and recovery.

Tennis pro Novak Djokovic attributes his success in recent years to a change of diet. He's won six of his seven Grand Slam tournament championships since adopting a "performance-focused" gluten-free diet.

Pole vaulter Jenn Suhr won the gold medal at the 2012 Olympics after switching to a gluten free diet.

Swimmer Dana Vollmer, brought home two Olympic gold medals she too is gluten free.

The Tour de France Garmin Team switched to gluten free to reduce inflammation.

And the Los Angeles Lakers' basketball team has changed their diet. They now eat organic grass fed meats, low carbohydrates, organic vegetables, and low-sugar foods. They avoid carbohydrates and processed foods. Lakers trainer Gary Vitti said,

"It wasn't an easy sell," Kobe Bryant was really on board right away because, as he's getting older, he knows he needs an edge and that nutrition can be one of them. Since he's adopted it, he says he feels remarkably better."

Bryant has credited the diet of lean meat and vegetables, and avoiding carbohydrates, especially sugar, with his remarkable late-career resurgence.

If this attention to diet can help professional athletes think what it can do for you. Try it for a week and then a month and then it will become a part of your life.

Exercise

Start exercising. Exercising not only makes your body healthier and much better looking it will help in treating fatigue. How?

After exercising, you will feel more energized. Exercise gets your blood circulating and increases oxygen throughout your body. It will also increase your levels of growth hormones.

Exercise helps regulate your insulin levels. Your body releases endorphins the feel good hormone during exercise.

Water

Dehydration may cause fatigue so drink plenty of water.

Water helps to remove harmful toxins from our body, which are known to contribute to some illnesses and fatigue.

So, avoid dehydrating yourself by keeping a bottle of water handy wherever you are. It's recommended that you drink at least 8 to 10 glasses of water a day in order for you to keep yourself well-hydrated throughout the day.

Sleep

Having enough sleep is another key to treating chronic fatigue. Most people need at least 6 to 8 hours of sleep a day in order to repair and restore their body. If you do get enough sleep, you will feel rested and feel more energized when you wake up in the morning.

To improve the quality of your sleep don't use caffeine after lunch. Never eat after 7:00 P.M. Keep your bedroom dark and don't put a television set in it.

Sleeping means that your brain needs to reach the REM stage of sleep. This is where your body truly relaxes and rejuvenates, so you will awake fully rested.

If you need to wake up at 6 in the morning and you want to have a minimum of 7 hours of sleep, you have to go to bed before 11 in the evening.

Getting even an hour less sleep than you need each night can leave you drowsy and unable to manage your daily routine.

There are many natural remedies you can take to help you sleep. Calms Forte is a homeopathic product that helps you quiet your mind so you can fall asleep. Melatonin may help you sleep. Visit a health food store or vitamin shop to see the number of herbal combinations for sleep.

Breathing

Breathing is another important factor to fight fatigue. A lot of people take in short and shallow breaths. This reduces the amount of oxygen taken in by your body and makes your lungs and heart work harder.

So, instead of taking in short and shallow breaths, try to

breath long and deep breaths. Inhale through your nose and exhale through your mouth.

Relax

Learning how to relax is one of the keys to treating adrenal fatigue. Try exercising or yoga. Deep breathing exercises are also good as well as meditation.

Miscellaneous

Sunshine will help increase energy levels. If it's winter time and there is a lack of sunshine in your area, use a full spectrum light.

Constant noise can sap your energy. Try earplugs or a white noise machine.

Depression can also cause fatigue. It's best to rule it out. Again check with your physician for help. If you are depressed there are many natural solutions you can try.

Alcohol depresses your central nervous system and acts as a sedative, making you tired for hours after consuming only a drink or two. It can also disrupt your sleep.

Another way to fight fatigue and stress is by varying your daily routine. Try to mix up your daily schedule a bit. And as much as possible, try to do something new in your daily life. Too much routine will get you bored, which can eventually lead to fatigue and stress.

Changes in your daily routine can be as small as taking another route on your way home from work or shopping in a different mall. Be creative and don't be afraid to try out something new.

Boredom can cause fatigue and a lack of energy. If boredom is the reason for your lack of energy, you can correct it by doing something, getting out and living.

Try to find some fun in your life. This will keep you laughing, which is proven to be a very effective energy booster. You should do some fun activities with your family and friends at least every week in order for you to keep yourself energized.

Read my book *57 Tips on Where To Meet The Opposite Sex* to find new ways to eliminate boredom and to discover many new ideas about things to do. In it you will discover many places to find and meet new friends.

Allergies

Allergies and food sensitivities may cause fatigue and low energy. Many people have sensitivity to dairy and gluten products. Remove them from your diet for a month and see if your fatigue disappears. A naturopathic doctor can help you find out if you are sensitive to any foods.

Whenever possible avoid prescription drugs. The side effect of many prescription drugs is fatigue. It's very hard to combat this type of fatigue. However changing your diet and adding supplements may help.

The raw materials needed to produce energy in the body are food (nutrients), water and oxygen. If you do not have sufficient energy and are free of illness then one of the inputs to the energy equation is missing.

Your food must supply all of the nutrients needed to produce energy. Eating processed, denatured foods will not supply the nutrients. It is imperative that you change your diet to provide your body with the necessary ingredients for energy production.

CHAPTER 2-VITAMINS AND MINERALS TO COMBAT FATIGUE

Your body needs some basic nutrients to produce energy. Ideally you should get them from your diet. But much of our food today is depleted of vitamins and minerals. To compensate, you should be supplementing your diet with vitamins and minerals.

Your cells produce, store and deliver energy to your body. Not wanting to get too technical here, let me talk about your cells. They have a membrane that surrounds them and protects them from invaders. The nucleus inside the cell is the brain that controls the cell.

Mitochondria are also found inside your cells. They produce the energy in all of your cells by controlling the chemical reactions to produce energy.

This energy is the chemical ATP. The mitochondria are sometimes described as "cellular power plants" because they generate most of the cell's supply of adenosine triphosphate (ATP), used as a source of chemical energy.

Mitochondria convert oxygen and nutrients into ATP. The less ATP in your cells the less energy you will have. One way to increase your energy is to increase your ATP levels.

In order to produce energy, your cells need various vitamins, minerals and nutrients. Your body doesn't store much ATP. It makes it when needed. Thus, your body needs all of the ingredients necessary to make ATP as it's required.

The Krebs cycle (citric acid cycle) consists of a complex series of chemical reactions in your body that generates energy from food. The Krebs cycle synthesizes food into cellular energy. The Krebs cycle is carried out within the mitochondria.

ATP is produced during the breakdown of glucose. The Krebs cycle is only one part of a series of stages that cells must create to produce energy.

All energy in your body comes from ATP. Chemical reactions can only occur if the required nutrients are present. Some vitamins are essential for the production of ATP.

Magnesium

Magnesium helps your cells turn glucose into ATP. It's used in over 300 chemical reactions in the body including the production and transport of energy.

Magnesium is essential for nerve and muscle function. It's involved in energy metabolism. It activates various enzymes that contribute to energy production. Magnesium increases your levels of endurance and exercise.

Many people have a magnesium deficiency from the over consumption of processed foods. Supplemental magnesium is often needed.

Vitamin B-12

Vitamin B-12 has long been used for fatigue. Injections of B-12 can increase your energy levels almost immediately. You can ask your doctor for vitamin B-12 injections.

When taken by mouth you should use the sublingual supplements.

B complex

The B-complex contains all of the B vitamins. These support your body in almost all of its functions. B vitamins are depleted during stress and lost during food processing. The B vitamins are essential for cellular energy production.

They are water soluble so they must be taken every day.

Iron

At one time it was widely advertised that you should use iron if you were fatigued because you had "iron poor blood." Iron helps your red blood cells carry oxygen to the cells.

Most of us have sufficient iron levels and taking more can cause damage. Before taking iron supplements get your iron levels tested. If you are a vegetarian you might not be getting enough iron in your diet.

Most post menopausal women do not need iron. If you are one of the few who could benefit from iron supplements get tested before and while taking supplements. Make sure your doctor recommends iron before you start taking it.

Many multivitamin supplements can be found without iron.

Pantothenic acid

Pantothenic acid is vitamin B5. It supports the adrenal gland. It helps in the conversion of fat and sugar to energy. It can help prevent fatigue.

Pantothenic acid is needed in the Krebs cycle for the production of acetyl Co-A. Acetyl Co-A is used by the body in energy production.

Most of us need more pantothenic acid in addition to our vitamin B complex.

Vitamin D3

Vitamin D is responsible for many functions in your body. Sun exposure is not a reliable way for most people to get vitamin D. Your doctor can test you to see if you need to take vitaminD3.

Our cells have special receptors for absorbing vitamin D. There are many benefits to taking vitamin D3. It's one of the most frequently recommended supplements for people with fibromyalgia and chronic fatigue syndrome. It helps support your immune function. It is critical for bone health, cellular replication, insulin production, and heart health.

Sulphur

Sulphur especially the homeopathic form can be used to increase energy levels. It improves cellular energy production and detoxifies your cells. It also helps your brain maintain its oxygen balance.

Malic acid

Malic acid helps the body with ATP production. Malic acid is both derived from food sources and synthesized in the body through the Krebs cycle. It's important to the production of energy in the body during both aerobic and anaerobic conditions.

Apples contain malic acid. Maybe that's where the old saying, "An apple a day keeps the doctor away" came from. Relatively small amounts of malic acid are required to increase mitochondrial energy production and ATP formation.

Magnesium can be chemically combined with malic acid to form dimagnesium malate. It is used to treat fibromyalgia and fatigue.

Iodine

Low iodine levels will affect your thyroid and make you tired. Stress also increases your need for iodine.

Seaweed can boost your iodine levels. Before taking iodine supplements get your levels checked and make sure you are taking the non toxic kind.

Remember supplements are not drugs and don't work immediately. You will have to try some of them for a month or longer before getting results. If one of these supplements does not work try something else.

There is nothing better than getting help from a nutritionally oriented doctor or naturopath. They will have all the newest information.

CHAPTER 3- HERBS THAT COMBAT FATIGUE

Always check with your physician before taking any herb, vitamin or supplement. Some nutrients and herbs may interact with medications.

The herbs listed here are generally regarded as safe in the prescribed dosages. I didn't include herbs or nutrients that contain caffeine. Caffeine may give you a temporary boost in energy but it is not long lasting.

Herbs have been used for centuries for healing. There are many herbs that can be used to reduce fatigue and increase energy.

Ginko Biloba

Ginko is an herb that enhances blood circulation and improves blood flow to the brain. Rats completed a maze with fewer errors after using Ginko Biloba. It's one of the most widely prescribed herbs in Europe. It's considered safe in the recommended dosages.

Ginseng

Ginseng is an adaptogen. It helps the body to adapt to stress. It's also a fatigue fighter. Athletes have been using ginseng to increase energy, recovery, stamina and performance.

There are 3 different kinds of ginseng.

Chinese ginseng is considered a rejuvenating tonic. It increases energy and supports the adrenal glands. It's said to increase your cells' ability to use oxygen as a fuel and help your muscles use glycogen. Athletes use it to increase performance and help lessen recovery time.

Siberian Ginseng has immune-regulating and adaptogenic properties. Siberian ginseng is used for fatigue, exhaustion and stress. As an adaptogen, Siberian ginseng helps patients adapt to stress.

Siberian ginseng increases energy levels. Athletes improved exercise duration, stamina and enhanced performance with Siberian ginseng.

American ginseng can aid in restoring energy levels and strengthening the adrenal glands.

Ginseng is not a fast acting herb. It may take a month or longer for you to see results.

Ashwagandha

Ashwagandha, sometimes called Indian ginseng, has been used for centuries in India. It's an herb used to treat exhaustion. It reduces cortisol levels. It's a general tonic and adaptogen that helps the body adapt to stress.

Ashwagandha has been reported to increase DHEA levels.

Licorice root

Adrenal exhaustion which causes fatigue and lack of energy can be helped with licorice root. It has been used as a tonic and has a rejuvenating effect.

Rhodiola

Rhodiola is a plant used in traditional medicine in Eastern Europe and Asia to enhance physical and mental performance. It has been used since 77 A.D.

Rhodiola is an adaptogen that helps glycogen synthesis in muscles and muscle recovery after exercise.

Schizandra

Schizandra is widely used as a tonic in Chinese medicine. It is used to increase mental and physical endurance. The schizandra berry has been used for thousands of years in the Chinese culture.

It will increase energy at a cellular level and increases the nitric oxide level in your body. It's used to fight fatigue.

Astragalus

Astragalus is used as an herbal treatment for physical exhaustion. It is considered an energy tonic, used to treat fatigue.

Maitake

Maitake a mushroom is used in traditional Chinese and Japanese medicine to enhance the immune system. It has shown promise in fighting chronic fatigue.

Olive leaf extract

Olive leaf extract (Olea europea) has energy promoting properties.

You can make tea from any of these herbs and sip on it throughout the day. Always check with your physician before taking herbs. And again herbs are not fast acting, it may take a month or longer to see results.

CHAPTER 4- NUTRACEUTICALS

Whether you are running a marathon, just trying to find the energy to exercise more often or trying to get through the day, there are nutraceuticals and dietary supplements that will help you.

Nutraceutical is defined in Canadian law as referring to "a product isolated or purified from foods that is generally sold in medicinal forms not usually associated with food."

Need more energy? To get more get-up-and-go you must maximize your energy production in the mitochondria of your cells. The mitochondrial are known as the energy generators of the cell or the power factories of your cells.

Mitochondria play a critical role in producing energy. About ninety-five percent of cellular energy comes from the mitochondria. To keep your mitochondria healthy there are many nutrients that are needed.

The four nutrients you definitely should add are magnesium, D-ribose, L-carnitine and CoQ10.

D-Ribose

D-ribose is a simple sugar that can boost muscle energy. It begins the process for ATP production and is an essential component of energy production. You need D-ribose to produce and regulate ATP. It's found in all cells of your body.

D-ribose helps to fortify the mitochondria. It supports recycling of energy and rebuilds the cellular energy pool. Ribose regulates how much energy we have in our bodies.

It can help you to quickly restore energy levels. Athletes have been using it to enhance energy, improve exercise performance and for faster muscle growth. Brewers yeast is rich in d-ribose. D-Ribose is well tolerated.

There are many studies involving D-ribose. One such study proposed:

"As D-ribose has been shown to increase cellular energy synthesis in heart and skeletal muscle, study was done to evaluate if D-ribose could improve symptoms in fibromyalgia and/or chronic fatigue syndrome patients." (2)

The conclusion was that "D-ribose significantly reduced clinical symptoms in patients suffering from fibromyalgia and chronic fatigue syndrome.

"D-ribose resulted in a significant improvement in energy; sleep; mental clarity; pain intensity; and well-being, as well as an improvement in patients' global assessment. 66% of patients experienced significant improvement with an average increase in energy of 45% and an average improvement in overall well-being of 30%." (2)

Pyruvate

Pyruvate is part of the body's energy producing cycle, the Krebs cycle. Pyruvate helps to provide energy to cells.

The body produces pyruvate and D-ribose converts to pyruvate. The complex cycle of producing energy converts glucose to pyruvate to ATP.

There are numerous medical studies on the benefits of pyruvate.

This following study was performed on rats. "When provided as an oral supplement for several days, pyruvate enhanced aerobic endurance capacity." (3)

L-Carnitine

L-Carnitine is an amino acid. It helps to transport long-chain fatty acids into the cells to make energy. Long chain fatty acids are used to provide energy in the body. It also helps get energy to the heart.

L-carnitine helps the breakdown of fats in the mitochondria. It increases the use of fat as an energy source by transporting fatty acids into the mitochondria. L-carnitine plays a fundamental role in energy production.

Overweight people have trouble with the transport of fats in the body. L-carnitine assists the body with the use of fats for energy.

Red meat is a rich source of L-carnitine. L-carnitine may benefit endurance athletes and long distance runners.

There are numerous medical studies on L-Carnitine.

Acetyl-L-carnitine

Acetyl-L-carnitine or ALCAR, is an acetylated form of L-carnitine. ALCAR is superior to L-carnitine in terms of bioavailability.

ALCAR has the ability to cross the blood–brain barrier and enter the brain, where it acts as a powerful antioxidant.

Acetyl-L-carnitine can help increase energy production in the mitochondria. Many studies have been conducted on a combination of ALCAR and alpha lipoic acid. One study on rats has excited researchers.

"ALCAR+LA partially reversed the age-related decline in average mitochondrial membrane potential and significantly increased hepatocellular O(2) consumption, indicating that mitochondrial-supported cellular metabolism was markedly improved by this feeding regimen. ALCAR+LA also increased ambulatory activity in both young and old rats; moreover, the improvement was significantly greater in old versus young animals and also greater when compared with old rats fed ALCAR or LA alone."(4)

Another study concluded that: "Our data show that administering ALC may reduce both physical and mental fatigue in elderly and improves both the cognitive status and physical functions." (5)

And another study concluded: "ALCAR prevented ATP depletion; therefore, ALCAR may mediate its protective effect by buffering oxidative stress and maintaining ATP levels."(6)

The studies on ALCAR and alpha lipoic acid are numerous.

In other words, ALCAR and alpha lipoic acid increases energy, supports mitochondria and reduces fatigue. ALCAR is well tolerated.

The discussion from the Proceedings of the National Academy of Science U S A. Feb. 2002 sums it up:

"We demonstrated that feeding old rats ALCAR

markedly improves the average mitochondrial membrane potential, a key indicator of mitochondrial function, to a level no longer significantly different from that of young rats.

"Thus, LA may act synergistically with ALCAR to improve both fatty acid and glucose catabolism and energy production. Indeed, we have previously shown that LA alone also increases oxygen consumption and mitochondrial membrane potential, although not as effectively as ALCAR.

"Supplementing the diet of old rats with ALCAR + LA significantly improves many of the most frequently encountered age-related changes in mammals—namely loss of energy metabolism, increased oxidative stress, decreased physical activity, and as impaired cognitive function." (4)

Amino acids

Amino acids are the building blocks of proteins. They are made up of carbon, hydrogen, oxygen, and nitrogen.

L-carnosine increases muscle strength and endurance. Creatine supports short bursts of high-energy exercise.

Glutamine is involved in more metabolic processes than any other amino acid. Glutamine is converted to glucose when more glucose is required by the body as an energy source. Glutamine assists in maintaining the proper acid/alkaline balance in the body.

Glutamine is an amino acid used in protein synthesis. It's an energy source for the brain and can increase your stamina.

Isoleucine belongs to a special group of amino acids called branched-chain amino acids, which are needed to help maintain and repair muscle tissue. Leucine and valine are two branched-chain amino acids.

Isoleucine is needed for hemoglobin formation and also helps to maintain regular energy levels.

Isoleucine is important for stabilizing and regulating blood sugar and energy levels. It must be obtained through our diet as our bodies cannot produce it.

Tyrosine is an amino acid that is used by the cells to synthesize protein. It's used to increase energy production and reduce fatigue. Low levels of tyrosine contribute to fatigue.

Citrulline malate is an amino acid used to help increase energy.

Beta-Alanine is an amino acid. A study concluded, "Similarly, beta-alanine supplementation has been shown to delay the onset of neuromuscular fatigue.

"Beta-alanine supplementation seems to be a safe nutritional strategy capable of improving high-intensity anaerobic performance."(7)

Bee pollen

Bee pollen is used by many athletes to help recovery and stamina. Athletes report that bee pollen helps them exercise harder and helps them to recover more quickly.

Bee pollen contains many different nutrients. It may be used to treat fatigue. It can cause an allergic reaction.

DHEA

DHEA is a hormone secreted by the adrenal glands. DHEA levels decline as we age. Studies have shown it increases energy levels. Since it is a hormone you should consult your physician before taking it.

Glandulars

Glandulars are used to support your glands. A few of the glandular products you can buy are adrenal, thyroid, liver, pancreas, thymus and pituitary glandulars. Most come from purified animal glands. Thyroid and adrenal glandulars support energy levels. Again consult your doctor before taking any glandulars.

Phosphatidylserine

Phosphatidylserine helps with mental fatigue and supports your adrenal glands. It also improves the movement of nutrients into the cells. Phosphatidylserine enables your brain cells to metabolize glucose.

DMG

Dimethylglycine (DMG) enhances oxygen utilization and helps metabolism. It is needed for many biochemical reactions.

The Russians have been studying DMG for years. They have found that it fights fatigue and helps with mental clarity.

Athletes use it as a performance enhancer and to maintain high energy levels.

NADH

Nicotinamide adenine dinucleotide (NADH) is a critical part of the Krebs cycle and is used by your cells to produce ATP. NADH occurs naturally during the body's production of energy. It improves mental clarity, alertness, concentration and athletic endurance.

It has been used in treating chronic fatigue. NADH is found in meat, fish, and poultry.

CoQ10

Coenzyme Q10 helps your cells mitochondria make energy. Statin drugs deplete your CoQ10 levels. If you are taking statin drugs ask your doctor about supplementing with CoQ10.

CoQ10 helps provide the heart with the energy and the oxygen it needs. It helps the body fight free radical damage and fight fatigue.

CoQ10 is essential for cellular energy production. CoQ10 is an enzyme which is found naturally in your cells and mitochondria. It regulates the oxidation of fats and sugars into energy. It also stabilizes cell membranes.

Adrenal Tonics

Adrenal tonics and adaptogens help support the adrenal glands to enhance the body's energy level and fight off stress.

Adrenal fatigue is a major cause of fatigue and tiredness. Our body responds to stress by releasing hormones to help us deal with it.

However, if we subject our body to continuous stress, our adrenal glands become fatigued. Continuous stress causes the adrenals to produce hormones day after day and even hour after hour until they can't produce anymore.

With adrenal fatigue, you will feel excessively tired and you will be unable to concentrate. You will feel sleepy and your mind will be foggy.

If you suffer from adrenal fatigue, sleeping will not get your energy levels up. In fact, people with this condition feel that they need to sleep more even after they wake up in the morning. They feel like they didn't sleep at all.

Many people who suffer from adrenal fatigue don't get enough sleep, don't exercise, have too much stress and don't eat the right foods.

When we eat poorly and we go through extreme stress on a day to day basis, our adrenal glands will eventually become overwhelmed, which will result in the under production of hormones.

The adrenal glands become unable to keep pace with the constant stress of fight-or-flight. The adrenals control about 50 hormones, responsible for energy production.

Cortisol is released from the adrenals in response to stress. When the adrenal gland is working correctly and producing the proper amount of cortisol, the body can handle stress effectively.

If you want to boost your energy levels you must deal with adrenal fatigue. Learn ways to deal with the stress in your life. Learn how to reduce or eliminate stress. Meditation and relaxation exercises can help with stress.

Supplements for adrenal fatigue can help your adrenal gland function. Adrenal gland extract from bovine sources will help. Pantothenic acid will also help and it is found in most adrenal gland supplements.

If you think you have adrenal fatigue it would be worth your while to consult an integrative physician or naturopath. They can test for adrenal failure and prescribe the proper supplements.

Licorice root extract is used to improve the function of the adrenal glands.

The adrenal glands produce the hormones adrenaline, cortisol and DHEA to protect the body against stress.

Pregnenolone secreted by the adrenal glands is used to make steroid hormones. It is an energy enhancer. Consult a doctor before taking it.

Thyroid

Your thyroid gland regulates your metabolism. An underperforming thyroid will result in a lack of energy and fatigue. You should have your doctor check your thyroid levels. Your thyroid could either make too much hormone or not enough.

If it fails to make enough of the thyroid hormone it is called hypothyroidism. The symptoms include fatigue, cold hands and feet, constipation, dry skin and a hoarse voice.

Thyroid glandulars may help support your gland as will iodine, B vitamins, tyrosine and manganese. Kelp is a good source of iodine. Check with your doctor before using thyroid supplements.

The opposite occurs if the thyroid makes too much hormone and this is called hyperthyroidism. This too can cause fatigue, muscle weakness, weight loss, irritability and an increased heart rate. Glandulars won't help this condition.

Creatine

Creatine is a popular and widely researched natural supplement.

Creatine is involved in energy production. Athletes use it to increase performance and decrease muscle fatigue. It supplies energy to all of your cells. Fish and meats are good sources of creatine.

Creatine phosphate works to increase energy by supplying phosphate to recycle adenosine diphosphate (ADP) into ATP. When an ATP molecule releases energy it looses a phosphate. The energy molecule that has lost one phosphate is ADP or Adenosine Di-phosphate.

To get back to ATP a phosphate must be added. Creatine can donate the phosphate to the ADP molecule making it into ATP. (Again this is a very simple explanation of a complicated process.)

If the mitochondria are not efficient at converting ADP to ATP, your cells rapidly run out of energy. Consequently you are exhausted, fatigued, worn out and have no stamina. Your cells must rest before more ATP can be made. Creatine can help with this.

Creatine is stored in muscles and helps to generate

cellular energy for muscle contractions.

There are numerous medical studies on creatine.

Vinpocetine

Vinpocetine is derived from the periwinkle plant and widely used in Europe. It improves circulation within the brain and improves glucose utilization in the brain. It increases ATP.

Nucleotides

Nucleotides are molecules that form the structure of DNA and RNA. Nucleotides are essential to creating new cells. They are involved in energy production and metabolism.

They support energy, immunity and recovery when exercising. Nucleotides increase vitality and endurance. Some suggest that you should use a sublingual supplement for better results.

Nucleotides are available for horses. Now why would I mention that fact? Because horse trainers want products that work and they won't waste money on products that don't work. The other products readily available for horses are DMG, creatine, branch chain amino acids, taurine, and phosophatidylcholine.

A study on the effects of a nucleotide supplement on the immune and metabolic response to short term, high intensity exercise performance in trained male subjects showed:

"We concluded that a chronically ingested nucleotide supplement blunts the response of the hormones associated with physiological stress." (8)

A similar study concluded:

"This work suggests that a nucleotide supplement, given chronically may offset the hormonal response associated with demanding endurance exercise. Specifically, the body's reaction to the stress of training may be lessened." (9)

Nucleotides will aid in recovery from intense exercise, lessen stress and help with immunity.

Acetyl Co-A

The Krebs cycle takes glucose to pyruvate to acetyl Co-A to ATP. In view of this important reaction I wondered if acetyl Co-A was available as a supplement and would it survive the digestive system.

The acetyl Co-A supplements on the market are really precursors to acetyl Co-A. That is they contain the necessary nutrients in the proper ratios for your body to make acetyl Co-A but not acetyl Co-A itself.

The precursors are Calcium Pyruvate, Magnesium, Pantothenic Acid, Acetyl-L-Carnitine, and L-Cysteine. It's cheaper to buy the combination formula than to buy each nutrient separately.

ATP

You body stores energy in the ATP molecule. When energy is needed this molecule is broken down and energy is released.

ATP the energy molecule is available as a supplement. So why not forget all of the other things I've mentioned and go right to the final product? Take ATP and be done with it.

ATP will restore your energy levels almost immediately. The problem is that ATP can cause stomach problems and nausea. And according to the following study oral ATP is not absorbed.

"Oral ATP supplements have beneficial effects in some but not all studies examining physical performance. One of the remaining questions is whether orally administered ATP is bioavailable.

"A single dose of oral ATP supplement is not bioavailable, whether administered as proximal-release or distal-release enteric coated pellets, or directly instilled in the small-intestine. This may explain why several studies did not find ergogenic effects of oral ATP supplementation. Also, more studies are needed to determine whether chronic administration of ATP will enhance its oral bioavailability."(10)

Another study using enteric coating ATP seemed to contradict the above study and found that ATP benefited athletes.

"The collective findings of our current study suggest that oral supplementation with ATP in combination with high intensity, periodized RT, increases muscle mass, strength, and power compared with a placebo-matched control. Moreover, when faced with greater training frequencies, oral ATP may prevent typical declines in performance that are characteristic of overreaching."(10a)

Again this supplement is not readily available at health food stores but can be found on the web and in large vitamin shops. More studies are being conducted every year. I haven't tried oral ATP to know if it works or not. If you are going to try it use the sublingual tablets or the enteric coated tablets.

To increase your get-up-and-go you must increase your cellular energy. The four nutrients that are vital for increased vim and vigor are D-ribose, L-carnitine, CoQ10 and magnesium.

To summarize D-ribose is an essential component of energy production. L-carnitine increases your energy by burning fat within the cell. CoQ10 allows the transport of fatty acids into the cell. And magnesium is crucial for energy production.

Used together they will have a synergetic effect. You will find you have more get-up-and-go than before and feel better than ever.

CHAPTER 5 - DETOXIFICATION

Detoxification

Over time our bodies store heavy metals, pesticides, herbicides, toxins and chemicals. These contribute to low energy. These toxins can destroy your cells and overload your liver.

A detox allows the body to cleanse itself naturally, effectively eliminating toxins that are stored deep within the tissue and organs for optimal inner and outer health.

During a detoxification you may feel worse for a while due to the toxins being pulled from the cells.

Schedule a detoxification every change of season.

Modified Citrus Pectin

Modified citrus pectin (MCP) is a form of pectin that has

been altered so that it can be more easily absorbed by the digestive tract. Studies have shown that oral MCP supplements significantly increase urinary excretion of toxic metals present in the body.

MCP is used to bind molecules, such as heavy metals or minerals, and hold them tightly so that they can be removed from the body.

There are many studies on MCP's chelating effects. I will mention two such studies on the detoxifying effects of MCP.

"The investigators reported that significant urinary excretion of arsenic, mercury, cadmium, and lead increased within one to six days of MCP treatment. There was a 150% increase in the excretion of cadmium and a 560% increase in lead excretion on day six. Essential minerals such as calcium, zinc, and magnesium were not seen to increase in the urine analysis, indicating that MCP treatment did not deplete these nutrients"(11)

"Heavy metal body burden can contribute to chronic disease, as well as interfere with the body's capacity to recover from illness. The five case studies show that reduction in toxic heavy metals (74% average decrease) was achieved without side effects, with the use of PectaSol modified citrus pectin (MCP) alone or with an MCP/alginates combination." (12)

MCP is an effective chelator. Use it to cleanse your

body of heavy metals.

Cholerella

Cholerella is considered a super food. Chlorella is a genus of single-cell green algae. It will bind with heavy metals and take them out of the body. Cholerella is one of the few foods that contains all the amino acids.

Blue green algae and spriulina are algaes that can also detoxify harmful chemicals.

Japanese studies show chlorella's detoxification properties are due to both the chlorophyll content and the substances in the cell walls.

Alkaline Foods

Your body functions best when it is slightly alkaline. An acidic body will result in a lack of energy and fatigue.

Most of the foods we eat in the standard American diet are acidifying. Our diet of meat, refined carbohydrates, sugar, fast food, coffee, soda, and white flour is highly acidic.

Alkaline foods are fruits and vegetables. Most of us don't eat enough of these foods to neutralize surplus acids. Eating leafy green vegetables and fruits keep the body alkaline. Eating foods containing chlorophyll will help to alkalize the blood and prevent osteoporosis. Eighty percent of the foods you eat should be alkaline forming foods.

Increasing the alkalinity of your body will result in less fatigue and a greater feeling of well being. It will also make you healthier.

Baking Soda

Sodium bicarbonate (baking soda) can be taken as a supplement. It will buffer acid production in the body thus making it more alkaline.

One study showed that "Sodium bicarbonate ingestion has been shown to improve performance in single-bout, high intensity events, probably due to an increase in buffering capacity."(13)

It can cause stomach upset in large amounts.

Aqua flora

If your fatigue is caused by the yeast overgrowth of Candida, aqua flora may help. It has been used to eliminate Candida. Aqua flora is a homeopathic remedy.

Other ways to help rid the body of yeast are first to eliminate all sugars from your diet. Yeast thrives on sugar. Take a good probiotic. Caprylic acid, oil of oregano, garlic, taheebo tea, and grapefruit seed extract can be used to help rid the body of yeast.

Garlic

Garlic is another herbal detoxifier. Sulfur containing

herbs help to detoxify your body.

Flor Essences

Flor Essences is a gentle, deep-cleansing herbal tea that detoxifies your cells.

Flor Essences consists of eight herbs: Burdock root, sheep sorrel herb, slippery elm bark, watercress, Turkish rhubarb root, kelp, blessed thistle herb, and red clover blossom.

These herbs have been shown to cleanse, detoxify, strengthen, and heal your body. It's very gentle and you should notice results with one bottle.

CHAPTER 6 - MISCELLANEOUS

Acupuncture

Acupuncture is used for a variety of health problems including fatigue. It's used to balance the flow of Qi throughout the body.

Numerous studies show acupuncture is effective in fighting fatigue.

Cell salts

Cell salts are homeopathic remedies for various ailments. Kali Phos is a cell salt used for fatigue.

Gelsemium

Gelsemium is a homeopathic remedy that is used for fatigue. Homeopathic remedies have been used for centuries in Europe. Gelsemium is used for unrefreshed sleep, fatigue and muscle weakness.

Octacosanol

Octacosanol is found in wheat germ oil. It has long been used by athletes to improve exercise performance including strength, stamina, reaction time and to increase physical endurance.

Aromatherapy

Aromatherapy can also help you out when it comes to fighting fatigue. Try peppermint, eucalyptus, rosemary and jasmine essential oils, as these scents are know to be energizing.

Most essential oils are used externally. Essential oils can be used topically to increase and balance your energy.

You can try putting a few drops on the collar of your shirt or on a handkerchief to smell throughout the day.

NT Factor

NT Factor is formulation of phospholipids. These are fats that are building blocks of cell membranes.

NT Factor can reduce fatigue and increase mitochondrial function. There are many studies on NT Factors and energy.

One study concluded, "A 33% reduction in fatigue after eight weeks on the supplementation product. The average initial fatigue score for the group before treatment was reported as severe after four weeks rated moderate and at eight weeks rated as moderate.

"The average (mean) score improved 33% from the initial survey before taking PNTF. Age was not associated with the degree of change in fatigue. Summary scores showed women improving by 35% and men by 29%." (14)

Another study reported, "The dietary supplement with NTF reduced significantly moderate fatigue as measured by the Piper Fatigue Scale and significantly increased mitochondrial function in aged subjects.

"The score of moderately fatigued subjects was reduced 20.2%. Further use of NTF for a total of eight or twelve weeks decreased the overall average score of moderately fatigued subjects 33%. (15)

Maca root

Maca, a member of the mustard family, is found wild in Peru, Bolivia, Paraguay, and Argentina. Maca is used to relieve stress and regulate metabolism.

Athletes use maca to enhance energy, stamina and endurance. It's an adaptogen.

Huperzine A

Huperzine A is a substance purified from a plant called Chinese club moss. It increases alertness and energy.

Glucuronolactone

Glucuronolactone is a substance that is found in the human body. It is produced in the liver when glucose is metabolized. It's a common ingredient in energy drinks.

It is used to boost energy increase alertness and reaction time and detoxify the body.

NO

Nitric oxide (NO) is produced in your body. It increases energy. Beets are a natural source of NO. Athletes use beet juice before an event to increase their energy. NO is available as a supplement.

NO (Nitric Oxide) aids in regulating ATP levels.

Cordyceps

Cordyceps is a fungus that has a long history in Chinese medicine. Cordyceps increases energy, stamina and physical performance.

"This small pilot study shows a pattern of physiologic changes during incremental exercise testing that lends support to the hypothesis that Cs-4, the standardized fermentation product of naturally occurring C. sinensis, enhances aerobic performance in older human subjects. These findings support the belief, long held in China that Cordyceps sinensis has the potential to improve exercise capacity and resistance to fatigue." (16)

The objective of this next study: "To evaluate effects of CordyMax Cs-4, a mycelial fermentation product of

Cordyceps sinensis, on energy metabolism."

This study on mice had these results, "Steady-state beta adenosine triphosphate (ATP) increased in the liver of mice that received CordyMax (200 or 400 mg/kg per day) for 7 days, by 12.3% +/- 0.8% and 18.4% +/- 0.9%, respectively, compared to placebo controls (both $p < 0.001$).

"CordyMax is effective in improving bioenergy status in the murine liver, suggesting a mechanism underlying the known clinical effectiveness of CordyMax in alleviating fatigue and improving physical endurance, especially in elderly subjects." (17)

Alpha-ketoglutarate

Alpha-ketoglutarate is a chemical found in the body and part of the Krebs cycle. It increases nitric oxide in the body. It can improve peak athletic performance.

I looked for some studies on alpha-ketoglutrate and fatigue but couldn't find any. I did find some studies that showed it improved bench pressing.

CHAPTER 7 - WHAT TO DO- 5 STEPS TO ELIMINATE FATIGUE IN YOUR LIFE

Conclusions:

Are you overwhelmed by the list of energy supplements? I've been asked why not just give us one or two supplements that work instead of all of these.

Because every one of us is different, what you are deficient in might not be what I am deficient in. If magnesium works for you, you want to tell everyone. But I might have enough magnesium and be deficient in CoQ10. So I've listed as many of the energy nutrients as possible.

I've listed so many different supplements that it would be impossible to take them all not to mention cost prohibitive. So what should you do?

Always rule out any severe illness with a complete

physical exam by your family doctor. And remember to talk to your doctor about any of the supplements you will be taking.

The five steps to more energy naturally are:

1. First you must change your diet. Eliminate all whites from your diet. That is white flour, white sugar, white rice, and white bread. Eliminate simple sugars, alcohol, and processed foods. These are the foods that rob your body of energy. They are empty calorie foods. Optimal nutrition is the first step to more energy.

Add nutrient dense foods, lean meats, organic produce and whole grains.

This is the best step you can take. The sad fact is that for most of us it will take quite a bit of time to remove all the bad things from our diet and make the lifestyle choices that will increase our energy. Most of us can't wait that long to feel better. So start step one and continue on with step 2.

2. While eliminating the processed foods from your diet start to detoxify. Our environment is full of toxic chemicals and they find their way into our bodies. The best detox is a gentle one. I would recommend modified citrus pectin. The complex includes alginate which is seaweed that will help to bind the toxic metals and eliminate them from your body.

This detox will eliminate heavy metals from your cells.

It might take at least a month to see results. But it's a must to increase your energy levels.

3. The next step is to give your body the nutrients it needs to produce energy. Your body must produce thousands of chemicals in the right amounts and at the right time. Our diets are incomplete and our foods are grown in depleted soils. Thus supplementation, especially as we age, is necessary.

While waiting for the lifestyle changes and the detoxification to take effect take a good multi vitamin and B complex. Include vitamin D3. CoQ10 and magnesium are also needed.

4. To get more immediate results use D-Ribose. D-Ribose goes to work immediately in the body, fueling the mitochondria to produce ATP. It works rapidly and is definitely worth trying.

Your body needs D-Ribose to make ATP. D-Ribose will restore your energy quickly.

Don't ignore steps 1, 2 and 3 even if D-Ribose works for you.

5. For more energy use NT factors. Some people get immediate results with NT factor lipids. Others take a week or more to get results. Again the results can be impressive with this supplement.

This study concluded, "After 60 days use of a

supplement containing a mixture of phosphoglycolipids, CoQ10 and NADH, fatigue measured with the validated Piper Fatigue Scale was significantly reduced in 58 patients with chronic fatigue syndrome/myalgic encephalomyelitis, chronic Lyme disease or other fatiguing illnesses, such as fibromyalgia syndrome or Gulf War illness. The supplement was safe and effective and reduced overall fatigue 30.8% in these long-term patients with intractable chronic fatigue.

"The supplement product, ATP Fuel®, containing NT Factor®, microencapsulated NADH, CoQ10, pro and pre-biotics and other nutrients (Researched Nutritionals, Inc., Los Olivos, CA), is a patent-pending proprietary nutrient complex containing an exogenous source of polyunsaturated phosphatidylcholine, phosphatidyglyerol, phosphatidylserine, phosphatidylinositol, and other membrane phospholipids, as well as coenzyme Q10 (CoQ10), microencapsulated reduced nicotinamide adenine dinucleotide (NADH) and other micronutrients." (18)

This was an impressive study. It seems this combination would be worth looking into.

There are basically 3 ways to increase your energy. One is to supply your body with all the nutrients it needs to make ATP. The other is to keep the mitochondria healthy and NT Factors helps in that regard. And the last way would be to recycle ADP into ATP.

If I had to add another few supplements DMG, and creatine help in the recycling of ADP to ATP. A supplement that seems to be very promising is ALCAR with alpha lipoic acid.

I hope that one of these nutrients will be effective for you. May all your days be full of energy.

Always consult your physician before self medicating. For more information on supplements and nutrients for good health consult a naturopathic physician.

You can find a vitamin supplier for most of these supplements at the website http://www.thecenterforweightloss.com just click on any vitamin banner.

REFERENCES

1. Steven R. Gambert, MD. Fatigue: Finding the Cause of a Common Complaint. *Clinical Geriatrics* 2005.

2. Teitelbaum JE, Johnson C, St Cyr J. The use of D-ribose in chronic fatigue syndrome and fibromyalgia: a pilot study. *Journal of Alternative and Complementary Medicine*. Nov. 2006.

3. Ivy, John. Effect of pyruvate and dihydroxyacetone on metabolism and aerobic endurance capacity. *Medicine & Science in Sports & Exercise*. June 1998.

4. Hagen TM, Liu J, Lykkesfeldt J, Wehr CM, Ingersoll RT, Vinarsky V, Bartholomew JC, Ames BN. Feeding acetyl-L-carnitine and lipoic acid to old rats significantly improves metabolic function while decreasing oxidative stress. *Proc Natl Acad Sci U S A*. Feb. 2002.

5. Malaguarnera M, Gargante MP, Cristaldi E, Colonna V, Messano M, Koverech A, Neri S, Vacante M,

Cammalleri L, Motta M. Acetyl L-carnitine (ALC) treatment in elderly patients with fatigue. *Arch Gerontol Geriatr.* 2008 Mar-Apr;46(2):181-90.

6. Dhitavat S, Ortiz D, Shea TB, Rivera ER. Acetyl-L-carnitine protects against amyloid-beta neurotoxicity: roles of oxidative buffering and ATP levels. *Neurochem Res.* 2002 Jun;27(6):501-5.

7. Artioli GG, Gualano B, Smith A, Stout J, Lancha AH Jr. Role of beta-alanine supplementation on muscle carnosine and exercise performance. *Med Sci Sports Exerc.* 2010 Jun;42(6):1162-73.

8. Mc Naughton L, Bentley D, Koeppel P. The effects of a nucleotide supplement on the immune and metabolic response to short term, high intensity exercise performance in trained male subjects. *J Sports Med Phys Fitness*. 2007 Mar;47(1):112-8.

9. Mc Naughton L, Bentley DJ, Koeppel P. The effects of a nucleotide supplement on salivary IgA and cortisol after moderate endurance exercise. *J Sports Med Phys Fitness.* 2006 Mar;46(1):84-9.

10. Ilja CW Arts, Erik JCM Coolen, Martijn JL Bour1, Nathalie Huyghebaert, Martien A Cohen Stuart, Aalt Bast and Pieter C Dagnelie. Adenosine 5'-triphosphate (ATP) supplements are not orally bioavailable: a randomized, placebo-controlled cross-over trial in healthy humans. *Journal of the International Society of Sports Nutrition* 2012, 9:16

10a. Jacob M Wilson, Jordan M Joy, Ryan P Lowery, Michael D Roberts, Christopher M Lockwood, et.al. Effects of oral adenosine-5'-triphosphate supplementation on athletic performance, skeletal muscle hypertrophy and recovery in resistance-trained men. *Nutrition & Metabolism* 2013, 10:57

11. Isaac Eliaz, Arland T. Hotchkiss, Marshall L. The effect of modified citrus pectin on urinary excretion of toxic elements. *Phytotherapy Research*. Oct. 2006.

12. Eliaz I, Weil E, Wilk B. Integrative medicine and the role of modified citrus pectin/alginates in heavy metal chelation and detoxification--five case reports. *Forsch Komplementmed*. Dec. 2007.

13. Lindh AM, Peyrebrune MC, Ingham SA, Bailey DM, Folland JP Sodium bicarbonate improves swimming performance. *Int J Sports Med*. 2008 Jun;29(6):519-23. Epub 2007 Nov 14.

14. Rita R. Ellithorpe, MD, Robert A. Settineri, MS, Garth L. Nicolson, PhD. Reduction of Fatigue by Use of a Dietary Supplement Containing Glycophospholipids. *The Journal of the American Nutraceutical Association*. 2003 Vol. 6 No. 1, 2003, 23-28.

15. Michael Agadjanyan, PhD, Vitaley Vasilevko, PhD. Nutritional Supplement (NT Factor™) Restores Mitochondrial Function and Reduces Moderately Severe Fatigue in Aged Subjects. *The Journal of Chronic Fatigue Syndrome*. 2003. 11(3): 23-36

16. Steve Chen, M.D., Zhaoping Li, M.D., Ph.D., Robert Krochmal, M.D., Marlon Abrazado, B.S., Woosong Kim, B.S., and Christopher B. Cooper, M.D. Effect of Cs-4® (Cordyceps sinensis) on Exercise Performance in Healthy Older Subjects: A Double-Blind, Placebo-Controlled Trial. *J Altern Complement Med.* 2010 May; 16(5): 585–590.

17. Dai G, Bao T, Xu C, Cooper R, Zhu JS. CordyMax Cs-4 improves steady-state bioenergy status in mouse liver. *J Altern Complement Med.* 2001 Jun;7(3):231-40.

18. Garth L. Nicolson, Robert Settineri, Rita Ellithorpe. Lipid Replacement Therapy with a Glycophospholipid Formulation with NADH and CoQ10 Significantly Reduces Fatigue in Intractable Chronic Fatiguing Illnesses and Chronic Lyme Disease Patients. *International Journal of Clinical Medicine*. Vol.3 No.3(2012).

RESOURCES

http://www.lindatremer.com
http://www.thecenterforweightloss.com
http://www.funwhilelearning.com
http://www.landbproducts.com

If you looking for some good children's books check out Jenny Lillystone on Amazon.com under books.

L & B Products has a fine line of kitchen and outdoor products.

ABOUT THE AUTHOR

Linda Tremer is a wellness coach. She has been studying and writing about health and natural medicine for over 25 years. She has written many articles for the website http://www.thecenterforweightloss.com.

You can visit her website http://www.lindatremer.com

She has written 2 fiction books:

The Persistent Ghost – An inspirational book for teens and adults.

Food to Die For – A mystery novel about the dangers of genetically modified foods.

She has written 3 non-fiction books:

Happiness Is A State of Mind

57 Tips on Where To Meet the Opposite Sex

How to Increase Your Energy Naturally

Her new non-fiction book *Refuse To Lose* should be available soon.

She has written children's books under the name Jenny Lillystone.

Fast Animals

Logging

And the military series:

Military Cargo Planes

Military Amphibious Vehicles

Military Heavy equipment

Armored Military Vehicles

http://www.funwhilelearning.com

All books are available at Amazon